BATTLING MYASTHENIA GRAVIS

A Beginners Guide To Myasthenia Gravis: Diagnosis, Treatment, Coping & Living Well

ROGER ANDREW

Contents

Introduction 4

CHAPTER ONE 9

Anatomical And Physiological Study Of The Neuromuscular Junction 9

Reasons And Threat Factors 15

CHAPTER TWO 21

Indications And Symptoms 21

Diagnostic Techniques 27

CHAPTER THREE 37

Medications Used To Treat Myasthenia Gravis...37

Experiencing Myasthenia Gravis 46

CHAPTER FOUR 56

MG Management Throughout Pregnancy 56

Conclusion..64

THE END 69

Introduction

Myasthenia gravis (MG) is a chronic autoimmune neuromuscular disorder that primarily affects the voluntary movement-controlling muscles. The condition is characterized by fatigue and muscle weakness that worsen with activity and improve with relaxation. The term "myasthenia gravis" derives from the Greek for "grave muscle weakness."

Here is how MG operates:

• Myasthenia gravis is an autoimmune disorder in which the immune system erroneously targets and attacks the acetylcholine receptor (AChR) or other proteins involved in nerve-muscle communication at the neuromuscular junction. Neuronal signals from motor neurons stimulate muscle contractions at the neuromuscular junction.

• Impaired Nerve-Muscle Communication: In a healthy neuromuscular junction, nerve signals release the neurotransmitter acetylcholine (ACh), which binds to ACh receptors on the membranes of muscle cells, causing muscle contractions. In myasthenia gravis, the autoimmune attack damages or reduces the number of ACh receptors on the membrane of muscle cells, thereby impeding the transmission of nerve signals to the muscles.

• Muscle Weakness: Due to impaired nerve-muscle communication, the muscles receive fewer signals from the nerves, resulting in muscle weakness, particularly during repetitive or prolonged activities. Eyelid lowering (ptosis), double vision (diplopia), difficulty swallowing (dysphagia), and generalized muscle weakness are typical MG symptoms.

• MG is characterized by fluctuating symptoms, with muscle weakness getting worse with activity and getting better with relaxation. This variation in symptoms can make diagnosing MG difficult.

• There is no cure for myasthenia gravis, but there are several treatment options available to manage the condition and alleviate symptoms.

These treatments may include cholinesterase inhibitors, immunosuppressive medicines, and plasma exchange or intravenous immunoglobulin (IVIG) treatments. In severe cases, surgical interventions such as thymectomy (thymus gland excision) may be advised.

The severity and progression of MG can differ from individual to individual. Many people with myasthenia gravis can lead relatively normal lives and obtain good symptom control with the proper treatment.

Individuals with MG must work closely with healthcare professionals, such as neurologists and immunologists, to develop a personalized treatment plan that addresses their specific requirements.

CHAPTER ONE
Anatomical And Physiological Study Of The Neuromuscular Junction

The neuromuscular junction (NMJ) is a specialized synapse or connection site between a motor neuron and a skeletal muscle fiber.

It serves a vital role in the communication between the nervous and muscular systems, allowing for voluntary muscle contractions. The neuromuscular junction's anatomy and physiology involve a number of essential components and processes.

The neuromuscular junction's anatomy:

• A motor neuron is a nerve cell that derives from the central nervous system (usually the spinal cord) and extends its axon to innervate skeletal muscle fibers. These neurons are responsible for electrical signal transmission to muscles.

• Axon Terminal: The extremity of the axon of a motor neuron is composed of numerous axon terminals or synaptic terminals. Each axon terminal establishes a synaptic connection with a single muscle fiber.

3.The synaptic cleft is a minute space separating the axon terminal of the motor neuron from the muscle fiber. It is the location where the nerve and muscle communicate.

• A muscle fiber, also known as a muscle cell or a muscle fiber cell, is a long, cylindrical cell that composes skeletal muscles. At its neuromuscular junction, a single motor neuron innervates each muscle fiber.

• Motor End Plate: The motor end plate is a specialized region of the sarcolemma (cell membrane) of the muscle fiber that is directly opposite the axon terminal. It contains a high concentration of acetylcholine receptors, which are necessary for nerve signal transmission to muscle fibers.

Neuromuscular Junction Physiology:

• Nerve Impulse Transmission: When a motor neuron receives a signal to initiate a muscle contraction from the central nervous system, it generates an action potential, an electrical signal that travels down its axon.

• When the action potential reaches the axon terminal, the neurotransmitter acetylcholine (ACh) is released from vesicles stored in the axon terminal. The ACh in the synaptic cleft is released.

• ACh binds to receptors on the motor end plate of the muscle fiber's sarcolemma. This binding activates ACh receptors, resulting in a localized change in membrane potential called an end-plate potential (EPP).

• Action Potential Generation: The EPP induces an action potential in the sarcolemma of the muscle fiber. Through a network known as the T-tubule system, this action potential then propagates along the muscle fiber's membrane and deep into the muscle fiber.

• Calcium ions (Ca2+) are released from the sarcoplasmic reticulum, a specialized organelle in muscle cells, when the action potential extends to the sarcoplasmic reticulum. Calcium ion release initiates the sliding filament mechanism, which leads to muscle contraction.

- Termination of ACh Action: The enzyme acetylcholinesterase, which breaks down ACh in the synaptic cleft, terminates the action of acetylcholine. This precludes continuous stimulation of the muscle and permits relaxation.

The neuromuscular junction is essential for voluntary muscle control, allowing the nervous system to precisely initiate and regulate muscle contractions. Any disturbance in this process can result in neuromuscular disorders, such as myasthenia gravis, or impaired muscle function.

Reasons And Threat Factors

Myasthenia gravis (MG) is primarily an autoimmune disorder, meaning it is caused by the immune system attacking the neuromuscular junction. It is believed that a combination of genetic, environmental, and immunological factors contribute to the development of multiple sclerosis (MG). Here are some myasthenia gravis-related causes and risk factors:

• Autoimmune Response: The development of autoantibodies against specific components of the neuromuscular junction is the most significant factor contributing to MG.

In the majority of instances, these autoantibodies target the acetylcholine receptors (AChRs) on the membrane of muscle cells or other proteins involved in nerve-muscle communication, thereby interfering with the transmission of nerve signals to the muscles.

• Genetic Factors: Although MG is not inherited directly, evidence suggests a genetic predisposition. Some individuals' susceptibility to developing the condition may be increased by genetic factors. It is more prevalent in families with a history of autoimmune diseases.

• Abnormalities of the thymus gland: The thymus gland, which plays a role in the maturation of immune cells, is frequently linked to MG. In some patients with MG, the thymus organ may be abnormally large or contain thymomas, which are tumors. Surgical removal of the thymus (thymectomy) can sometimes alleviate symptoms, especially in younger people.

• Certain environmental factors, including viral infections (e.g., Epstein-Barr virus), have been suggested as potential triggers for MG in genetically predisposed individuals. These infections may stimulate the immune system and result in the development of autoantibodies.

• Myasthenia gravis affects people of all ages, but is more prevalent in women under the age of 40 and men over the age of 60.

• People with other autoimmune diseases, such as lupus, rheumatoid arthritis, or Hashimoto's thyroiditis, may be at an increased risk for developing MG. This suggests that a common underlying immune dysregulation may be present.

• Certain medications, such as certain antibiotics, muscle relaxants, and antihypertensive drugs, can exacerbate MG symptoms or precipitate a myasthenic crisis (a abrupt deterioration of muscle weakness).

• Stress and Fatigue: Although stress, physical fatigue, and emotional fatigue are not primary causes of MG, they can exacerbate its symptoms.

Not everyone with these risk factors will develop myasthenia gravis, and the precise cause varies from person to person.

MG is typically diagnosed and treated using a combination of clinical evaluation, antibody testing, and other diagnostic procedures to determine the underlying cause and determine the most effective treatment. Typically, treatment options concentrate on enhancing neuromuscular transmission and suppressing the autoimmune response.

CHAPTER TWO
Indications And Symptoms

Myasthenia gravis (MG) is characterized by muscle weakness and fatigue, especially in the voluntary muscles, which are the muscles you can control consciously. The severity and specific symptoms of MG can vary from patient to patient, but common symptoms include:

1. Muscle Weakness Muscle weakness is the defining symptom of myasthenia gravis. It typically begins in the ocular (eye) muscles and can spread to other muscle groups.

Common signs and symptoms include:

• Drooping eyelids (ptosis) can impair vision if one or both eyelids descend.

• Double vision (diplopia): Individuals with MG may perceive a single object as two separate images.

• Ingesting difficulty (dysphagia): Chewing and ingesting food or liquids can become difficult.

• Facial muscle weakness can result in a "mask-like" facial expression.

• Muscular weakness in the neck can make it challenging to hold the head up.

2. Muscle Fatigue: Muscle weakness in MG frequently intensifies with repeated or prolonged muscle use. Reading, speaking, and chewing may become problematic after a brief period of time due to muscle fatigue. Resting typically provides temporary relief from fatigue.

3. In severe cases of MG, respiratory muscles can weaken, resulting in breathing difficulties. This condition is potentially fatal and requires urgent medical attention.

4. Weakness of the Limbs and Trunk: MG can affect the muscles of the limbs, legs, and trunk. Lifting objects, walking, and ascending stairs may become more difficult.

5. Changes to the Voice Weakness in the muscles responsible for speech (dysarthria) can result in changes to the voice, such as a nasal or distorted speech pattern.

6. Difficulty with Activities of Daily Living: MG can impair a person's ability to carry out daily activities such as dressing, holding objects, and sustaining balance.

7. MG is characterized by fluctuating symptoms throughout the day, which is one of its defining characteristics. Symptoms may be exacerbated by physical exertion and alleviated by rest.

8. Bulbar symptoms can include difficulties with chewing, swallowing, and speaking. Bulbar symptoms involve muscles associated with the mouth and esophagus.

9. Paradoxically, after a period of rest, some individuals with MG experience an increase in muscle weakness. This condition is referred to as "post-rest fatigue."

10. Sensory and Pain Symptoms: Although uncommon, some individuals with MG may experience sensory and pain symptoms.

It is crucial to note that the severity of MG varies from person to person, with some experiencing mild symptoms that affect only a few muscle groups, while others experience more extensive muscle weakness.

MG symptoms can vacillate over time, alternating between periods of improvement (remission) and worsening (relapse). A healthcare professional, typically a neurologist, can help individuals with MG effectively manage their symptoms and maintain a high quality of life through prompt diagnosis and treatment. Treatment options may include neuromuscular transmission-enhancing medications, immunosuppressive drugs, thymectomy (thymus gland removal), and supportive care.

Diagnostic Techniques

Myasthenia gravis (MG) is typically diagnosed through a combination of clinical evaluation, specialized diagnostics, and medical history evaluation. Due to the fluctuating character of its symptoms and the need to distinguish it from other neuromuscular disorders, MG can be difficult to diagnose. Here are some common diagnostic procedures and assays for MG:

1. Medical Background and Physical Exam:

• A thorough medical history is required, including a discussion of symptoms, their onset and progression, as well as any factors that worsen or alleviate symptoms.

• A comprehensive physical examination, including a neurological assessment, can help identify muscle weakness, eye abnormalities (such as ptosis or diplopia), and other clinical signs of MG.

2. The Tensilon (Edrophonium) Test:

• The Tensilon test entails intravenous administration of the drug edrophonium (Tensilon). Edrophonium temporarily inhibits the breakdown of acetylcholine (ACh), thereby increasing ACh concentrations at the neuromuscular junction.

• Individuals with MG typically experience a temporary increase in muscle strength, particularly in the ocular muscles, following the test. This improvement is typically temporary (lasting only a few minutes) and serves to corroborate the diagnosis.

3. Electromyography (EMG) consists of the following

• Electromyography measures electrical muscle activity. The response to nerve stimulation is recorded after a special needle electrode is inserted into the muscles and the response to nerve stimulation is recorded.

• Muscle atrophy and fatigue may be observable via EMG in MG due to repetitive nerve stimulation.

4. Blood Exams:

• Specific antibodies associated with MG can be detected by blood tests. The most frequently examined antibody is anti-acetylcholine receptor antibody (anti-AChR).

• The anti-muscle-specific kinase (anti-MuSK) antibody is a frequently tested antibody. Some individuals with MG lack anti-AChR antibodies and instead have this antibody.

• Blood tests may also be used to evaluate other variables, such as thyroid function, in order to rule out conditions that can mimic MG symptoms.

5. SFEMG: Single Fiber Electromyography:

• SFEMG is a more sensitive test for detecting abnormalities in neuromuscular transmission. It measures the latency and jitter (variability) of muscle fiber responses to nerve stimulation.

• It can be especially helpful in diagnosing MG when conventional EMG results are ambiguous.

6. Imaging Research:

• The thymus organ can be examined using imaging techniques such as computed tomography (CT) and magnetic resonance imaging (MRI). Some instances of MG are associated with thymic abnormalities, including thymomas and thymic hyperplasia.

7. PFTs (Pulmonary Function Tests):

• Pulmonary function tests, such as spirometry, can evaluate lung function and assist in detecting respiratory muscle paralysis in severe cases of myasthenia gravis.

8. Ice Pack Exam:

• An ice compress may be applied to the eyelids of a person with ptosis in certain instances. If the ptosis resolves temporarily, this may indicate MG.

9. Test of Repetitive Nerve Stimulation (RNS):

• RNS involves repeatedly stimulating a nerve with electrical impulses while measuring muscle responses. In MG, repetitive stimulation results in a characteristic diminution (reduction) of muscle response amplitude.

10. Serological Examines:

• Antibodies against AChR or MuSK in the blood can be detected using serological tests, such as enzyme-linked immunosorbent assay (ELISA).

MG is frequently diagnosed through a combination of these tests and a thorough clinical evaluation. The choice of diagnostic tests may vary according to the individual's symptoms and the healthcare provider's clinical judgment.

To enhance the quality of life for individuals with MG, early diagnosis and appropriate treatment are essential. Once a diagnosis has been made, treatment options can be tailored to the patient's specific requirements in order to manage symptoms and lessen the impact of the condition.

CHAPTER THREE
Medications Used To Treat Myasthenia Gravis

Myasthenia gravis (MG) symptoms are effectively managed with the aid of medication. The purpose of treatment is to enhance neuromuscular transmission, reduce muscle weakness, and lessen the influence of the disease on daily life.

Typically, the selection of medication and dosage is based on the individual's unique requirements and the severity of their symptoms.

The following medications are commonly used to treat MG:

1. Cholinesterase Blockers:

• Cholinesterase inhibitors, such as pyridostigmine (Mestinon) and neostigmine (Prostigmin), are frequently the first-line treatment for multiple sclerosis (MG).

• They function by inhibiting acetylcholinesterase, an enzyme that degrades acetylcholine (ACh) at the neuromuscular junction. These pharmaceuticals enhance muscle stimulation by increasing ACh levels.

• Cholinesterase inhibitors are especially useful for treating ptosis, diplopia, and muscle paralysis.

• Dosing is individualized and based on the patient's response and symptoms.

2. Immunosuppressive Pharmaceuticals:

• Immunosuppressive pharmaceuticals are used to inhibit the autoimmunity that attacks the neuromuscular junction. Typically, these medications are prescribed to patients with moderate to severe MG.

• Prednisone, azathioprine (Imuran), mycophenolate mofetil (CellCept), and cyclosporine are common immunosuppressive medications.

• These medications decrease inflammation and the production of autoantibodies, thereby stabilizing or ameliorating MG symptoms over time.

• Immunosuppressive therapy frequently necessitates routine monitoring of blood counts and other possible adverse effects.

3. The corticosteroid hormones:

• Corticosteroids, such as prednisone, are occasionally used to treat MG symptoms, particularly in severe cases.

• They function by inhibiting the immune response and diminishing inflammation.

• Due to the possibility of side effects, corticosteroids are frequently combined with other immunosuppressive medications.

4. IVIG: Intravenous Immunoglobulin.

• Individuals with swiftly worsening MG symptoms or those who cannot tolerate other therapies may be treated with IVIG.

Immunoglobulin (antibodies) obtained from pooled blood donations are administered intravenously. IVIG is capable of modulating the immune response.

• The effects of IVIG are typically temporary, and treatment may require periodic repetition.

5.   Exchange   of   Plasma (Plasmapheresis):

• Plasma exchange entails the removal of the patient's blood plasma (which contains the detrimental antibodies) and its replacement with a substitute, such as albumin or fresh frozen plasma.

• This procedure decreases the concentration of autoantibodies and can temporarily alleviate MG symptoms.

• Plasma exchange is a common treatment for severe conditions, including MG crises.

6. Antibodies that are Monoclonal:

• Rituximab and eculizumab are monoclonal antibodies that target specific immune cells or proteins that contribute to the immune response. They may be considered for patients who do not respond to alternative therapies.

• Rituximab targets B cells, which are responsible for producing the autoantibodies that attack ACh receptors.

• Eculizumab inhibits the complement system, which contributes to immune-mediated injury.

7. The thymectomy:

• Individuals with MG may undergo surgical removal of the thymus gland (thymectomy), particularly if they have thymomas (tumors in the thymus gland) or thymic hyperplasia.

• Thymectomy can reduce or eliminate MG symptoms in some cases, particularly in younger patients.

The choice of medication or combination of medications for the treatment of MG depends on the patient's specific symptoms, response to treatment, and potential adverse effects. Individuals with MG must work closely with neurologists and immunologists to develop a personalized treatment plan and undergo routine monitoring to optimize symptom management and quality of life.

Experiencing Myasthenia Gravis

Myasthenia gravis (MG) can affect numerous aspects of daily life, making it challenging to live with the condition. However, many individuals with MG are able to live fulfilling lives with the appropriate management and support. Here are some living with MG advice and considerations:

1. Medical Administration:

• Seek advice from a neurologist or neuromuscular specialist with experience treating MG. Regular follow-up appointments are necessary to monitor your condition, modify your medications, and evaluate the efficacy of your treatment.

• Comply with your prescribed medication schedule. Take medications as prescribed by your doctor, and promptly report any adverse effects or concerns.

• Maintain a symptom journal to monitor changes in your condition, which can be useful during doctor's visits.

2. Behavioral Modifications:

• Prioritize rest and pacing: Myasthenia gravis symptoms frequently worsen with exertion, so it is essential to manage your energy levels. Plan to prevent excessive fatigue by limiting your leisure time.

• Avoid triggers: Identify and reduce aggravating factors that worsen your symptoms. This may include exposure to tension, extreme temperatures, and specific medications.

• Make a plan for assistive devices: Depending on the severity of your muscle impairment, you may benefit from mobility aids, speech aids, or adaptive tools to assist with daily activities.

3. Diet and nourishment:

• Ensure a balanced diet: Maintain a nutrient-dense diet and consult a registered dietitian for individualized dietary recommendations. Adequate nutrition can aid in muscle maintenance and overall health.

• Swallowing issues: If you have trouble swallowing (dysphagia), work with a speech therapist and a dietitian to develop safe and nutritious feeding strategies.

4. Physical activity and Physiotherapy:

• Engage in low-impact exercises, such as walking, swimming, or tai chi, that are appropriate for your condition. Physical therapy may be useful for maintaining muscle function and stamina.

• Consult your healthcare provider or physical therapist for advice on an appropriate, individualized exercise regimen.

5. Support Method:

• Establish a support network: Inform your peers and family of your MG diagnosis to help them comprehend your condition and provide emotional support.

• Join a support group: Interacting with others with MG can provide valuable insights, advice, and emotional support. There are numerous support organizations available online and in local communities.

6. Mental Health and Adjustment:

• Due to its impact on daily activities, MG can be emotionally trying. Consider seeking assistance from a therapist or counselor if you are experiencing stress, anxiety, or depression to help you endure.

• Learn relaxation techniques: Techniques for stress management, such as deep breathing, mindfulness, and meditation, may reduce symptom exacerbation.

7. Safe Driving Practices:

• Consult your healthcare provider if you experience significant muscle weakness that impairs your ability to drive safely. You may need to modify your driving habits or, in extreme cases, cease driving temporarily.

• Ensure the safety of your living environment to avoid accidents caused by muscle weakness.

8. Strategy for MG Crises:

• Recognize the symptoms of a myasthenic crisis (severe muscle weakness that impairs respiration) and have an emergency plan in place. This may include knowing when to seek immediate medical care and having access to contact information for emergency services.

9. Discuss your condition with your employer to investigate workplace accommodations, such as modified work hours, ergonomic adjustments, or telecommuting, if applicable.

10. Represent Yourself:

• Advocate actively for your own health. Inform yourself about MG, ask questions during doctor visits, andtinănature-second opinions.

• Remain current on the latest MG research and treatment options.

The fluctuating nature of MG necessitates ongoing management and adaptation. By working closely with healthcare providers, maintaining a supportive network, and making lifestyle adjustments, many individuals with MG can lead fulfilling lives and achieve excellent control over their symptoms.

CHAPTER FOUR
MG Management Throughout Pregnancy

Myasthenia gravis (MG) requires cautious planning and coordination between you, your healthcare providers, and specialists during pregnancy.

Pregnancy can have a substantial impact on MG symptoms, and it is crucial to prioritize both the mother's health and the fetus's development. Here are some factors to consider and management strategies for MG during pregnancy.

1. Preconception Preparation:

• If you are contemplating pregnancy, you should consult with your healthcare provider, preferably a neurologist or neuromuscular specialist, prior to conception. This enables for a thorough evaluation of your MG condition and any necessary medication adjustments.

2. Medication Administration:

• Your healthcare professional may need to modify your MG medications before or during pregnancy. Due to potential hazards to the fetus, it may be necessary to modify or discontinue the use of certain medications used to treat MG.

• Discuss your current medication regimen, potential hazards, and alternative treatment options with your healthcare provider. The objective is to minimize the impact on the developing infant while managing your MG symptoms effectively.

3. Frequent Observation:

• Maintain close contact with your healthcare provider throughout your pregnancy. Your MG symptoms, muscle strength, and medication demands will be monitored more frequently than usual.

• Prenatal visits should also include monitoring the baby's growth and well-being on a regular basis.

4. Expert Care Groupa:

• Assemble a team of healthcare professionals with experience managing MG during pregnancy, including a neurologist, obstetrician, and potentially a specialist in high-risk pregnancies (maternal-fetal medicine specialist).

• Open communication: Ensure that your healthcare providers collaborate and communicate effectively to provide you with individualized, comprehensive care.

5. Lifestyle Administration:

• Prioritize rest: Fatigue can exacerbate MG symptoms, so ample rest and pacing are essential during pregnancy.

• Maintain a well-balanced diet to support your overall health and the health of your child. Consult with a dietitian if necessary.

• Gentle exercise: Participate in pregnancy-appropriate mild, low-impact exercises, such as prenatal yoga or swimming, as approved by your healthcare team.

6. Be Aware of Volatility:

• MG symptoms may vacillate during pregnancy, with some individuals experiencing improvement and others experiencing deterioration. Prepare for and communicate these changes to your healthcare provider.

7. Prenatal Planning:

• Develop a birth plan with your obstetrician and neurologist, taking your MG symptoms and potential labor and delivery complications into account.

• It is essential to have a pain management plan in place, as certain pain medications can affect MG symptoms.

8. Neonatal Graves Myasthenia (NMG):

• Infants born to mothers with MG may be at risk for developing neonatal myasthenia gravis, though the condition is typically temporary and self-limiting. Prepare yourself for possible monitoring and treatment of your child.

9. After Birth Care:

• Your MG symptoms may vacillate again after delivery. Ensure that you have a system of support in place to assist with infant care and daily activities.

Management of MG during pregnancy requires a team approach and cautious monitoring to strike a balance between the mother's health and that of the unborn child.

Your healthcare providers will collaborate with you to create a personalized care plan that addresses your unique requirements and ensures the best possible outcome for you and your baby. Throughout pregnancy and the postpartum period, regular communication and collaboration with your medical team are crucial.

Conclusion

Myasthenia Gravis (MG) is a complex autoimmune neuromuscular disorder that causes muscle weakness and lethargy by affecting the neuromuscular junction. It's caused by the immune system's attack on specific neuromuscular junction receptors.

Although the precise cause is unknown, genetics, environmental stimuli, and thymus gland abnormalities can all contribute to its development.

MG is diagnosed through a combination of clinical evaluation, specialized diagnostics, and a review of the patient's medical history. The Tensilon test, electromyography, blood tests to detect specific antibodies, and imaging investigations are common diagnostic methods.

The treatment for MG emphasizes on symptom management and minimizing the disease's impact on daily life. To enhance neuromuscular transmission and suppress the autoimmune response, cholinesterase inhibitors, immunosuppressive medications, and monoclonal antibodies are frequently used. Additionally, surgical interventions such as thymectomy may be contemplated.

Living with MG requires adjusting to the fluctuating symptoms of the condition and managing energy levels. Lifestyle modifications, including adequate rest, a balanced diet, and gentle exercise, are essential aspects of self-care.

Individuals with MG can also improve their quality of life by constructing a support network, seeking emotional support, and addressing mental health issues.

For pregnant women with MG, careful planning and coordination with healthcare providers are required to ensure the health of both the mother and the developing embryo while managing the condition.

Individuals with MG can live fulfilling lives with proper medical management, support, and self-care techniques, despite the fact that the condition can present challenges.

MG patients have reason to aspire for improved outcomes and quality of life due to advances in treatment and ongoing research.

THE END